THALLASSEMIA

INTO ALL IT TAKES TO HEAL

THALLASSEMIA

DR. CYRIL LAKES

Contents

CHAPTER ONE

INTRODUCTION

Less hemoglobin and red blood cells than usual are the hallmarks of thallassemia, an inherited blood condition. There are various forms of thalassemia, such as Mediterranean anemia, Cooley's anemia, beta-thalassemia intermedia, and alpha-thalassemia.

The component of your red blood cells that enables them to carry oxygen is called hemoglobin. Thalassemia's low hemoglobin and fewer red blood cells can lead to anemia, which wears you out.

In cases of mild thalassemia, therapy might not be necessary. If your thalassemia is more severe, however, you might require frequent blood transfusions. Additionally, you can manage your weariness on your own by following a nutritious diet and getting regular exercise.

Symptoms of thalassemia include:

Weary

Deficiency

pale appearance

Skin discolouration that is yellow (jaundice)

abnormalities of the facial bones

gradual expansion

stomach edema

dark urination

The kind and degree of your thalassemia determine the indications and symptoms you encounter. While some infants may exhibit thalassemia symptoms from birth, others may experience them throughout the first two years of life. Some individuals with only one mutated hemoglobin gene do not show any symptoms of thalassemia.

If you are concerned about your child's signs or symptoms, schedule an evaluation with your child's physician.

Reasons

Mutations in the DNA of the cells that produce hemoglobin, the component of red blood cells that transports oxygen throughout your body, are the cause of thalassemia. Children inherit the thalassemia-related mutations from their parents.

The thalassemia-causing mutations impair normal hemoglobin production, resulting in low hemoglobin levels and a high rate of red blood cell loss, which ultimately leads to anemia. You feel exhausted when you have anemia because your blood doesn't have enough red blood cells to deliver oxygen to your tissues.

Thalassemia types

The amount of gene mutations you received from your parents and the portion of the hemoglobin molecule that is impacted by those mutations determine the type of thalassemia you have. Your thalassemia will be more severe if you have more mutated genes. The alpha and beta components of hemoglobin molecules are subject to mutation.

Thalassemia alpha

The production of the alpha hemoglobin chain involves four genes. Your parents each give you two. In the event that you inherit:

You won't have any thalassemia symptoms or indicators if there is only one faulty gene. However, you are a disease carrier and may infect your offspring.

Your thalassemia signs and symptoms will be minor due to two faulty genes. Alpha-thalassemia minor is the term used to describe this illness, or you may be told that you have alpha-thalassemia trait.

Your indications and symptoms will range from moderate to severe due to three faulty genes.

Hemoglobin H disease is another term for this illness.

The illness known as hydrops fetalis or alpha-thalassemia major is caused by four faulty genes. Usually, it results in the death of the newborn soon after birth or the fetus dying before delivery.

Thalassemia beta

The beta hemoglobin chain is made up of two genes. Your parents each give you one. In the event that you inherit:

With just one faulty gene, you'll only experience minor symptoms. This disorder is known as a beta-thalassemia trait or beta-thalassemia mild.

Your indications and symptoms will range from moderate to severe due to two faulty genes. Also referred to as Cooley's anemia, this illness is recognized as beta-thalassemia major. Typically, babies with two faulty beta hemoglobin genes are healthy at birth, but within the first two years of life, they start to show symptoms. With two faulty genes, a milder type known as beta-thalassemia intermedia may also arise.

RISK ELEMENTS

The following are some factors that raise your risk of thalassemia:

Thalassemia in the family history. Parents can pass on thalassemia to their offspring by way of altered hemoglobin genes. You can be more susceptible to thalassemia if there is a family history of the illness.

specific lineage. People with Italian, Greek, Middle Eastern, Asian, and African ancestry are most likely to have thalassemia.

COMMITMENTS

The following are potential thalassemia side effects:

Iron excess. The condition of thalassemia itself or repeated blood transfusions can cause an excess of iron to build up in the bodies of those who have it. Your heart, liver, and endocrine system which includes glands that create hormones that control bodily functions can all be harmed by an iron overload.

infection. Infection risk is higher in thalassemia patients. This is particularly true if you have undergone splenic removal.

bone abnormalities. Your bones may enlarge due to bone marrow expansion brought on by thalassemia. This may lead to aberrant bone structure, particularly in the skull and face. In addition to making bones brittle and thin, bone marrow growth raises the risk of shattered bones.

CHAPTER TWO

Spleen enlargement (splenomegaly). The spleen aids in the body's defense against infection and removal of undesirable substances, such as stale or broken blood cells. A huge number of red blood cells are frequently destroyed as a result of thalassemia, which causes your spleen to work harder than usual and grow. Splenomegaly can shorten the survival of red blood cells that have been transfused and exacerbate anemia. Your spleen could need to be removed if it becomes too large.

reduced rates of growth. A youngster may experience slowed growth due to anemia.

Thalassemia may also cause a delay in puberty in some youngsters.

cardiac issues. Severe beta thalassemia may be linked to cardiac issues, including arrhythmias and congestive heart failure.

Getting Ready for Your Consultation

Within the first two years of life, people with moderate to severe types of thalassemia are typically detected. See your pediatrician or family physician if you have observed any of the thalassemia signs and symptoms in your child. A physician who specializes in blood diseases, known as a hematologist, may then be recommended to you.

Being well-prepared is a good idea because appointments are often short and there is a lot of territory to cover. Here are some preparation tips and things to anticipate from your physician.

What you're capable of

Note any symptoms that you or your child are having, even if they don't seem to be connected to the reason you made the visit.

Important personal details, such as significant stressors or recent life transitions, should be included. Find out from your relatives if there is a family history of thalassemia on both sides of the family, and inform your physician if there is.

Enumerate any drug you take, along with any vitamins and supplements.

Prepare a list of inquiries for your physician

Making the most of your time with your doctor can be achieved by creating a list of questions in advance of your visit. In the event that time runs out, prioritize your list of questions from most to least important. Some fundamental inquiries for your physician regarding thalassemia are as follows:

Which of these conditions, if any, best describes me or my child?

Exist any more potential reasons?

Which types of testing are required?

Which therapies are offered?

Which medical procedures would you suggest?

Which adverse effects are most frequently experienced with each treatment?

I have these other medical issues, or my child has. What is the best way to manage them jointly?

Are there any dietary guidelines to adhere to? Do I need to take any dietary supplements for myself or my child?

Are there any printed materials available for me to take, such brochures? Which websites would you suggest?

Do not be afraid to ask any more questions that come up during your session, in addition to the ones you have prepared for your doctor.

You'll probably be asked a lot of questions by your doctor. Being prepared to respond to them could buy you extra time to discuss any topics you'd like to cover in greater detail. Your physician might inquire:

Is there anyone in your family affected by thalassemia?

Where in the world was your family originally from?

When did you start to have these symptoms?

Do you always have symptoms, or do they come and go?

What level of severity do you have?

Do you see any improvement in your symptoms?

What seems to exacerbate your symptoms, if anything?

Exams and diagnosis

Within the first two years of life, the majority of children with moderate to severe thalassemia exhibit signs and symptoms. Blood tests may be used to confirm a diagnosis of thalassemia if your child's physician has suspicions about the condition.

Blood testing could show the following if your child has thalassemia:

a low red blood cell count

less than anticipated blood cells in red

red blood cells that are pale

Red blood cells with a range of sizes and forms

Under a microscope, red blood cells with an uneven distribution of hemoglobin give the appearance of a bull's eye.

Moreover, blood testing can be used for:

Check the iron level in your child's blood.

Analyze his or her hemoglobin levels.

To diagnose thalassemia or find out if someone has altered hemoglobin genes, do a DNA analysis.

<h2 style="text-align:center">Prenatal examination</h2>

To find out if a newborn has thalassemia and how serious it might be, testing can be done before to birth. The following tests are used to identify thalassemia in fetuses:

Samples from Chorionic Villus. A little portion of the placenta is removed for analysis during this test, which is typically performed during the eleventh week of pregnancy.

Amniocentesis. This test, which often involves collecting a sample of the fluid surrounding the fetus, is carried out during the sixteenth week of pregnancy.

Technology for assisted reproduction

A type of assisted reproductive technology may help parents with thalassemia or bearers of a faulty hemoglobin gene give birth to healthy children by combining pre-implantation genetic diagnostics with in vitro fertilization. The process entails taking a woman's mature eggs and fertilizing them in a lab dish with a man's sperm. Only embryos free of genetic flaws are implanted into the woman after being examined for genetic problems.

The kind and severity of your thalassemia will determine how you are treated.

How to treat mild thalassemia

With thalassemia, signs and symptoms are typically moderate, and little to no therapy is required. Sometimes, especially after surgery, after giving birth, or to assist manage difficulties from thalassemia, you may require a blood transfusion.

For iron overload, beta-thalassemia intermedia patients may require medical attention. While beta-thalassemia intermedia patients may not require blood transfusions, which frequently result in iron overload, they may have increased iron absorption through the digestive tract. Deferasirox (Exjade), an oral medicine, can assist in removing the extra iron.

Moderate to severe thalassemia treatments

For mild to severe thalassemia, possible treatments include:

regular transfusions of blood. Blood transfusions are frequently necessary for more severe cases of thalassemia, sometimes even every few weeks. Iron builds up in the blood after blood transfusions, which can harm your heart, liver, and other organs. You might need to take iron-removing drugs to aid in your body's removal of excess iron.

transplant of stem cells. In certain circumstances, severe thalassemia may be treated by a stem cell transplant, often known as a bone marrow transplant. You get extremely high dosages of medication or radiation therapy to kill your damaged bone marrow before receiving a stem cell transplant. After that, stem cell infusions from a suitable donor are given to you. But because these operations have significant dangers, including the possibility of death, they are often only performed on the sickest patients who have a sibling or other suitable donor available.

WAY OF LIFE AND DOMESTIC MEDICINE

Thalassemia is usually not preventable. Before you conceive or father a child, you should think about seeking advice from a genetic counselor if you have thalassemia or if you carry the thalassemia gene.

Adapting and providing assistance

Thalassemia can be difficult to manage. You don't have to work alone, though. See a member of your healthcare team if you have any questions or need advice. Enrolling in a support group could also prove advantageous. This kind of group can offer helpful knowledge as well as empathetic listening.

THE END